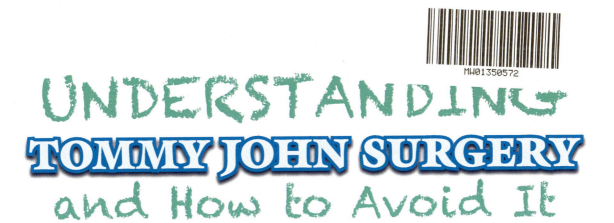

A Guide for Young Baseball Players

By Christopher S. Ahmad, MD, Frank Alexander, MS, ATC, Charles J. Ahmad

Lead Player LLC
New York
2017

© 2017 Lead Player LLC

All rights reserved. No part of this book may be reproduced in any form by any electronic or mechanical means (including photocopying, recording, or information storage and retrieval) without permission in writing from the publisher.

Printed and bound in the United States of America.

ISBN: 978-0-9963885-2-8

TABLE OF CONTENTS

Introduction 5

Chapter 1 : History of Tommy John Surgery 9

Chapter 2 : What is Tommy John Surgery? 15

Chapter 3 : Understanding the Elbow 21

Chapter 4 : What Causes Tommy John Injury? 23

Chapter 5 : Treatment of Tommy John Injury 29

Chapter 6 : How to Stay on the Field 33

Final Message from the Authors 38

Glossary 41

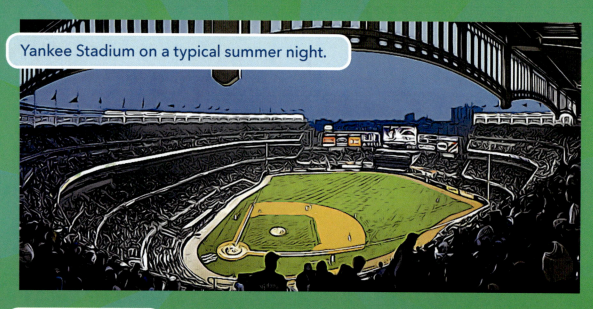
Yankee Stadium on a typical summer night.

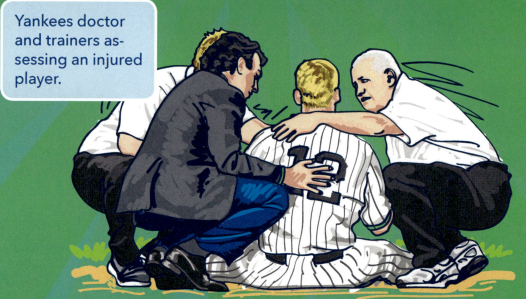
Yankees doctor and trainers assessing an injured player.

Introduction

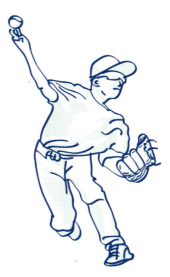

You're on the edge of your seat and sweating. The crowd around you hums, buzzes, and explodes with a roar at the pop of a blast deep to left field. Count one for the home team! It's the bottom of the 9th inning and you've got a hot dog in one hand and a glove resting on your lap. You're at Yankee Stadium on an early summer night—surrounded by fans, friends, and family. You hear mom and dad cheering for a home run, while others chant—"Strike! Strike! Strike!" The game is on the line. The pitcher wipes his forehead, adjusts his glove … and here comes the pitch!

Strike two hits the catcher's glove, but suddenly back on the mound, the pitcher is in terrible pain and holding his elbow against his body. Trainers rush to the mound wondering with everyone watching "What happened to his elbow? Will he be OK? Can he continue to pitch?"

These are the questions that Sports Medicine answers!

What is Sports Medicine?

Sports Medicine is an area of medicine where medical professionals care for injuries to the shoulder, elbow, knee, and other areas of the body that may be injured while playing sports. Sports Medicine professionals take care of all types of patients, not just athletes, and include:

Orthopedic (or·tho·pe·dic) **Doctors** take care of bones and joints such as the shoulder, elbow, and knee. You would usually go to a doctor's office to see them. These doctors can also be surgeons and perform surgery when necessary.

Nurse Practitioners (prac·ti·tion·ers), **Physician Assistants,** and **Nurses** can provide all-around care that helps get you back to feeling great and playing your sport.

Athletic Trainers are multi-skilled medical professionals that help prevent and care for sports injuries. Athletic trainers are often at games and practices and provide immediate care to an injured athlete.

Physical Therapists treat sports injuries using physical methods like targeted exercise, massage, and heat treatment.

> **Orthopedics** is a kind of medicine that treats the musculoskeletal (mus·cu·lo·skel·e·tal) system of the body, like the shoulder, elbow, knee, joints and ligaments, tendons, bones, and muscles.

Introduction

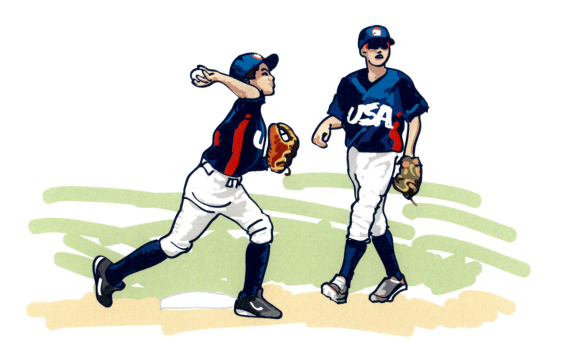

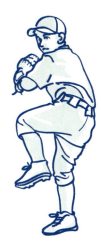

History of Tommy John Surgery

In 1974, there was a Major League Baseball Player named Tommy John who pitched for the Los Angeles Dodgers. On July 17th, 1974, Tommy had the best record in the League—13 wins and only 3 losses. On that day, he was leading the Dodgers to another victory, protecting a 4-0 lead. With a man on first base, Tommy John threw a pitch hoping for a double play and was surprised to feel a painful tearing sensation in his elbow. When asked, he could only describe it as "Somehow my arm was getting ripped from its socket."

The catcher caught the pitch and threw the ball back to the mound. Tommy tried throwing another sinker, but this time the ball sailed off-course, high up into the stands. With serious elbow pain, Tommy walked off the mound and immediately met with Dr. Frank Jobe in the trainer's room.

Dr. Jobe was the long time Team Doctor for the Dodgers, and trusted by the players when they got injured. He examined Tommy, performed x-rays, and told him that he had a torn **ulnar collateral ligament,** or UCL. Dr. Jobe treated Tommy with a cast on his arm. After a long period of rest, Tommy attempted to throw a baseball but was unable because of continued pain in his elbow.

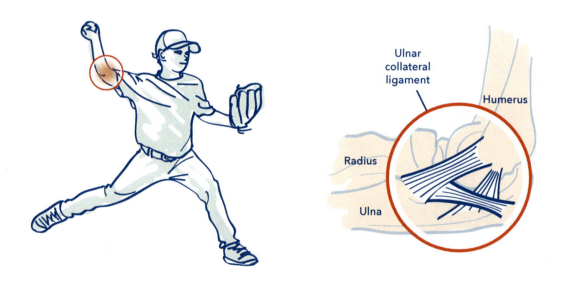

Throwing a baseball puts unnatural stress on the elbow.

Repetitive force can lead to swelling, microscopic tissue trauma, and tearing in the ulnar collateral ligament or the medial collateral ligament.

History of Tommy John Surgery

> The Ulnar collateral ligament is a thick triangle-shaped band at the inside part of the elbow uniting the humerus bone to the ulna bone. It consists of two portions, an anterior and posterior united by a thinner intermediate portion. The UCL is the most important ligament to a baseball player.

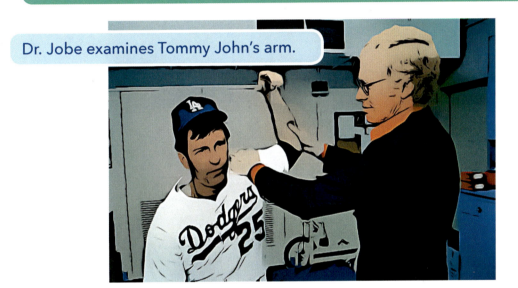

Dr. Jobe examines Tommy John's arm.

Making Baseball and Sports Medicine History

This was during a time when baseball players who injured their elbow UCL had to quit playing and give up on their dreams. Dr. Jobe told Tommy that his elbow injury did not heal, and he would have to quit playing baseball. Devastated, Tommy pleaded "Can't you fix my elbow with an operation?" Dr. Jobe explained that no operation existed that could fix his elbow. Tommy responded simply, "Well, make one then—I trust you." What happened next would forever link these two men, and change the history of baseball.

Dr. Jobe studied possible surgical methods to make a new ligament in Tommy's elbow, one that could get him back on the pitching mound. He finally invented a surgery that would rebuild Tommy's torn ligament by taking a tendon from his wrist and placing it in his elbow. Because of the complexity of the surgery and the surgery never having been done before, Dr. Jobe told Tommy he had a 1 in 100 chance of pitching again after the surgery. Without hesitation, Tommy said, "Let's do it." So, history was made, and Tommy John underwent the first ever UCL reconstruction surgery.

Tommy John Surgery Statistics

It is now estimated that 1 out of 4 professional baseball pitchers at the Major League level have had Tommy John Surgery. This number has been growing rapidly over the last several years. What is more concerning is that our younger athletes are getting injured even more rapidly than professional players. The majority of youth athletes that get injured are between the ages of 16 and 18 years old.

Do Other Athletes Get Tommy John Injuries?

Tommy John Injuries can occur in baseball players who play other positions such as catcher, outfielder, or infielder. Baseball players are not the only athletes that can get Tommy John Injuries. Athletes that compete in softball, gymnastics, tennis, volleyball, football, wrestling, and the track and field event of javelin—are also at risk for Tommy John Injury.

History of Tommy John Surgery

Javelin throwing puts force on the UCL and can cause UCL tears.

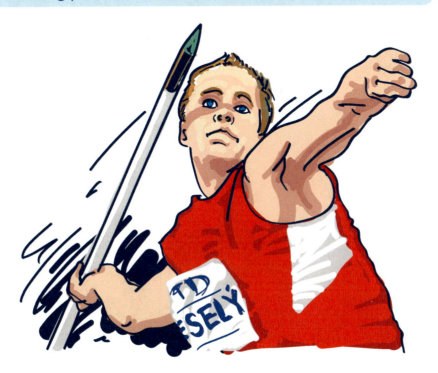

TOMMY JOHN SURGERY FACT:

The first torn UCL was diagnosed in a javelin thrower, not a baseball player!

CHAPTER 2

What Is Tommy John Surgery?

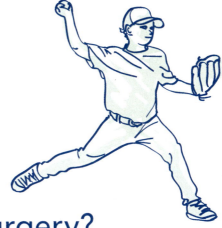

All baseball players can hurt their UCL, but it happens to pitchers most often. When a pitcher tears their UCL, they may feel:

- a pop in their elbow
- a tingling feeling in their pinky or ring fingers
- a tightness in their forearm

These are common symptoms, but not all players experience the same symptoms when they get injured. Once the UCL has a tear, the elbow hurts and players are unable to continue throwing.

> **Symptoms** are what a player feels that may mean an injury.

Understanding Tommy John Surgery and How to Avoid It

Pain on the inside part of the elbow may indicate a Tommy John Injury.

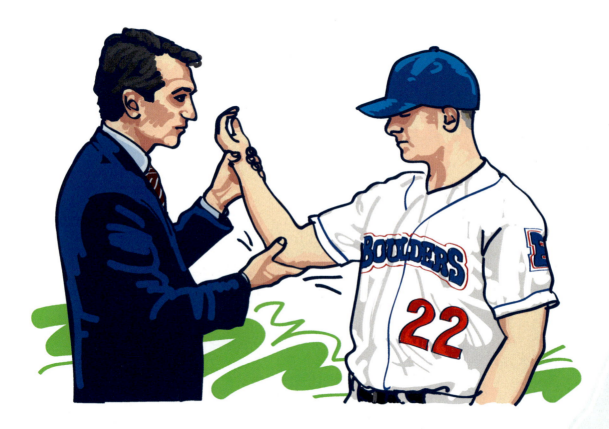

Moving Valgus Stress Test helps medical professionals see if a player has torn their UCL by applying pressure to the elbow.

SIGNS OF TOMMY JOHN INJURY

Early signs of an injury include:

- Loss of pitching velocity
- Loss of pitching control
- Feeling like it is hard to warm up
- Feeling elbow tightness
- Unable to fully flex or extend the elbow
- Swelling around the elbow
- Tingling sensation in the fingers

Late signs of an injury include:

- Pain on the inside part of the elbow when throwing
- Inability to play

Once a player develops symptoms of a UCL tear, an evaluation by their athletic trainer, doctor, or other medical professional should take place. If the symptoms develop during a game or practice, the athletic trainer is usually the first person to evaluate the player. The evaluation will include **palpation** (gently pushing) on the elbow and surrounding muscles and a special test called the **Moving Valgus Stress Test,** which will help the evaluator understand if the UCL has been compromised.

When the UCL is partially torn and not fully torn, many players are able to continue throwing—but say they do not throw as hard as they once did. Players may also say they are not as accurate as they used to be. After your athletic trainer has evaluated you, he or she may send you to an orthopedic doctor who specializes in baseball injuries.

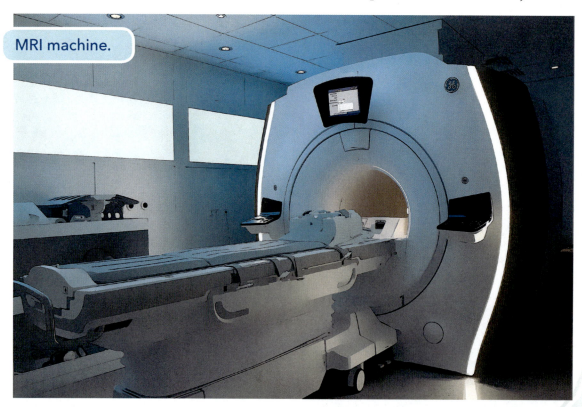

MRI machine.

Magnetic Resonance Imaging (MRI) is a way for doctors to look at pictures of your elbow. The MRI is like a giant magnet that is used with a computer to create pictures.

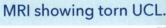

MRI showing torn UCL.

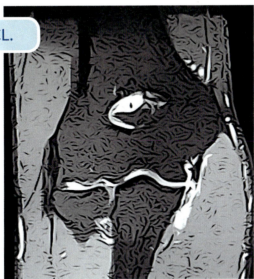

The doctor may send you to have an **Magnetic Resonance Imaging** (MRI) procedure. An MRI is used to evaluate the UCL and help tell the doctors and sports medicine staff if you have torn your UCL.

TOMMY JOHN SURGERY FACT:

1 in 4 Major League Baseball Pitchers have needed Tommy John Surgery. That's 25%!

CHAPTER 3

Understanding the Elbow

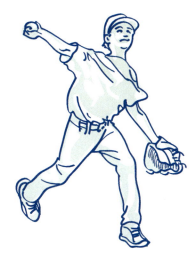

To understand more about Tommy John surgery and why baseball players get injured, we first need to look at the parts of the elbow and see its weaknesses. Our elbow is a joint that is considered a **hinged joint** that allows us to flex and extend our arms and legs.

> **Hinged Joint** refers to a common type that includes the ankle, elbow, and knee joints.

There are a few different parts of the elbow that are very important to baseball players—those are the **muscles, ligaments,** and **tendons** that make up our arms. Ligaments are similar to rope or string, and attach one bone to another bone. The ligament that attaches the bones of the elbow is called the ulnar collateral ligament, also known as the UCL. This ligament is put under a tremendous amount of force when throwing a baseball and can be injured or become torn. The ligament is similar in size to a shoe lace or Popsicle stick, and the length of an Oreo cookie.

CHAPTER 4

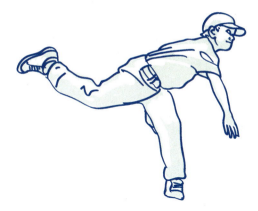

How Do Players Get the Tommy John Injury?

Nathan Learns Not to Ignore Pain

Nathan first felt elbow pain when he was 14 years old. He was pitching on 2 teams, and when he was not pitching—he was catching. He continued playing with pain, and didn't tell his parents because he was worried they would stop him from playing. One day Nathan felt so much pain with each throw that he had to tell his parents.

It was good that he did—they took him to visit the Team Doctor for the New York Yankees! The doctor examined his elbow and said he needed to have an MRI. The MRI scan pictures showed the UCL was completely torn. Nathan was devastated—treatment would need at least 4 months of down time, meaning no baseball. Rest would allow his UCL to heal. If it did not heal, it is likely Nathan would need Tommy John Surgery, which would mean an entire year without playing!

Why Are More Young Athletes Getting Hurt?

More and more pitchers are injuring their elbows than in previous years. In Major League Baseball, 25% of pitchers have already had Tommy John Surgery. Unfortunately, many players are now requiring a second Tommy John Surgery. Even more troubling is that younger athletes are now the group of baseball players who need Tommy John Surgery the most.

There are many reasons why baseball players tear the UCL. One major reason is overuse.

Most athletes want to play on as many teams and as many showcases throughout the year as possible, so coaches everywhere get to see them play. Sometime even scouts for colleges and professional baseball teams look for potential players at showcases. Playing in showcases will help a baseball player reach the next levels of play.

> **Overuse** is when a player throws too much over a period of time.

Rest, Pitch Counts, and Radar Guns

Trying to impress scouts and college coaches comes at a price. Without time to rest and recover from throwing, your elbow ligament can break down and tear. Think of your UCL ligament as a wire clothes hanger or a paper clip—the more you bend it back and forth, the weaker it gets until it eventually breaks.

Players may tear their UCL if they throw too many pitches in a single game. So it's really important to have a plan to limit your pitch count every time you play. If you play on multiple teams, you should set a pitch count that is suited to your schedule

How Do Players Get the Tommy John Injury 25

so you avoid injury. Keeping track of your pitches and innings thrown is a great way to monitor the stress on your arm. Even if your pitch count is low, if your elbow begins to hurt, you need to let your coach, parents, or caregiver know.

Pro Tip : Focus On Mechanics Over Speed

Many young players want to know how hard they throw, and so they ask their parents for a radar gun to find out. Radar guns are helpful at the more advanced level of play for many reasons, but for young athletes, trying to throw hard is not as important as having good pitching mechanics. When an athlete tries to throw hard, they're increasing the stress placed across the elbow joint, specifically across the UCL. Young athletes should focus on their mechanics, and less on speed. As players mature, velocity will follow more safely.

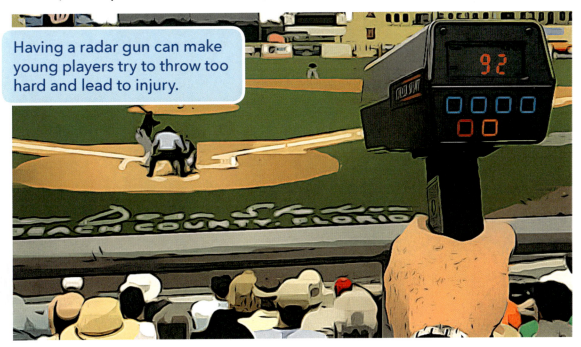

Having a radar gun can make young players try to throw too hard and lead to injury.

Fatigue and Early Specialization

Another reason a pitcher can injure their UCL is if they continue to pitch when tired. This is also known as fatigue. When a pitcher is fatigued, they will often make up for it with a change in their throwing mechanics. When a pitcher's mechanics are "off," there is an increased risk of injuring the UCL. Knowing when you are tired or when you've reached your limit will help you avoid an injury to your UCL.

> **TOMMY JOHN SURGERY FACT:**
>
> Tommy John played in the MLB for 26 seasons and won 288 games—164 wins came after his surgery!

Early specialization describes athletes who choose to solely play a single sport. In baseball, early specialization is one of the strongest reasons why players get injured. Athletes who only play baseball are 70 to 90% more likely to get injured when compared to children who play multiple sports. Baseball players injure their elbow and shoulder more than other types of athletes.

Early specialization in baseball is risky. Young athletes are subjected to intense competition. This often results in not enough rest, playing year-round, and playing on multiple teams. In addition, without playing other sports such as basketball or soccer, constant repetition of the same athletic movements often leads to injury.

3 out of 4 children quit sports because sports are no longer enjoyable or because they're injured.

Multiple sport participation leads to:

- Better overall motor skills and athletic development
- Longer playing careers
- Increased ability to carry skills to other sports
- Increased motivation, ownership of the sports experience, and confidence

Playing a diverse set of sports at a young age yields a better ability to make important decisions during games. Athletes able to "read the game" in one sport, are better at adapting to another, similar sport.

The Risk of Velocity

Science tells us velocity has a direct relationship with stress on the ulnar collateral ligament. So a pitcher who throws 99 mph has a much higher risk of injuring his ligament in comparison with a pitcher who throws 80 mph. The average Major League fastball was 90.8 mph in 2008. In 2013, it had reached 92 mph—with eight pitchers hitting 100 mph.

CHAPTER 5

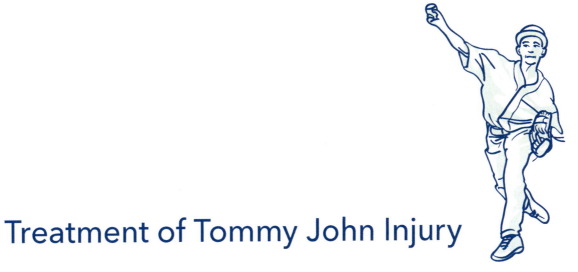

Treatment of Tommy John Injury

The main treatment for a Tommy John Injury is to stop throwing and allow time for the ligament to heal. This means no throwing baseballs or playing sports that resemble throwing, such as tennis. After several weeks of rest, players need physical therapy to strengthen their muscles before starting to throw again. It may take several months before getting back into a game.

Having Tommy John Surgery

When a player is not able to get healthy with rest and physical therapy, they will require Tommy John Surgery to repair the damaged UCL. To fix the ligament, an orthopedic doctor will take a tendon from another area of the body. This tendon is typically from the forearm or knee and is called a "graft". The new graft will take the place of the old, torn ligament.

> **Grafts** are pieces of living tissue that are moved from one part of the body to another through surgery.

Understanding Tommy John Surgery and How to Avoid It

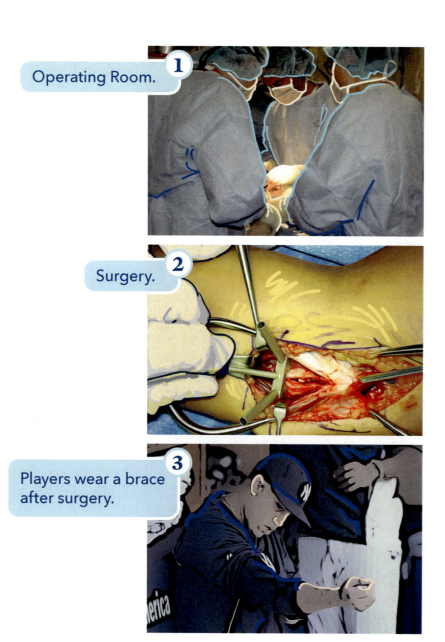

1. Operating Room.
2. Surgery.
3. Players wear a brace after surgery.

Treatment of Tommy John Injury

1. Surgeon making a skin incision over the inside part of the elbow.
2. Instruments helping surgeons perform Tommy John Surgery.
3. A player wearing a brace after surgery.

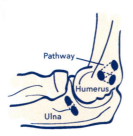

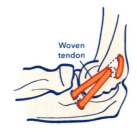

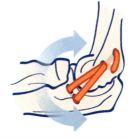

Typically, an orthopedic surgeon will drill pathways in the humerus and the ulna.

Tendon, harvested from the hamstring or forearm, is woven through the pathways in a figure-eight pattern.

The grafted tendon acts as a ligament, keeping the joint stable while anchoring the bones in place.

TOMMY JOHN SURGERY FACT:

Research has shown that 50% of baseball players have been encouraged to continue to play through pain.

CHAPTER 6

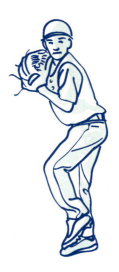

How to Stay on the Field

There are many ways that you can avoid an injury to your UCL, including:

Keeping a diary of how many innings and pitches you throw each week. This diary may vary week to week but helps you understand how much actual hard throwing you're doing.

Taking many breaks throughout the year. If you only play baseball, you especially need to give yourself breaks. This means that you do not participate in any baseball activity for a few weeks at a time. Our bodies need rest from the same sport.

During the season, making sure there is enough rest between the games. If you throw a lot in a game, make sure you're truly ready to play in the next one. Icing your arm will help keep any soreness at bay and will help your arm recover!

Training hard in the off-season. Training, or conditioning, in the off-season can help you strengthen your body in preparation for a long regular season.

Understanding Tommy John Surgery and How to Avoid It

TOMMY JOHN SURGERY FACT:

Research has shown that 75% of youth baseball players continue to play while experiencing elbow pain.

10 STEPS to PREVENT TOMMY JOHN SURGERY

1. Warm up properly.
2. Keep a diary of innings/pitches you throw.
3. Follow pitch counts.
4. Avoid playing on multiple teams.
5. Avoid pitching and playing another position during season.
6. Have a good off-season/in-season workout regimen.
7. Make sure you take at least 4 months from hard throwing off per year.
8. Play another sport in off season.
9. Ice your arm after each practice and game.
10. Don't play if you have arm pain!! Throwing with pain can be a cause of injury!

Know The Right Pitch Count

Pitch counts are the simplest way to manage overuse in baseball. Learn more about the appropriate pitch count here: **www.baseballhealthnetwork.com.** Pitchers should adhere to pitch counts and rest and avoid playing on multiple teams. If a pitcher is supposed to rest, he should not go to another team and pitch.

Baseball players should also be encouraged to play multiple positions. This decreases the likelihood of injury and enhances performance by improving understanding of the strategy behind each position to develop different skills. Playing another position has to be factored into their throwing volume. It avoids overuse of one set of muscles or joints to the point of injury.

The catcher is another important position with high throwing volume with the second highest risk of injury related to overuse. Encouraging players to rotate through different positions helps to rest certain muscle groups. Players should not play baseball more than 8 months in a year.

MISCONCEPTIONS

While Tommy John Surgery is on the rise, there are many myths that are NOT true, including:

- Tommy John Injuries and Surgery are inevitable.
- Tommy John Surgery will increase performance, such as increasing velocity.
- Tommy John Surgery is not related to overuse.
- The height of the pitcher's mound needs to be lower to decrease stress on the elbow.

The old saying is true—quality really is better than quantity when it comes to pitches. Throwing fewer pitches with greater concentration and body awareness does more for developing performance and talent than huge volumes of throwing. It's much better to learn how to throw strikes by developing movement on the ball than attempting to manage velocity and the amount of curve in curveballs.

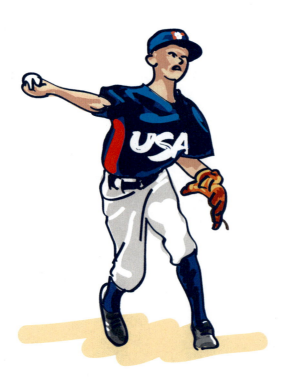

How to Stay on the Field 37

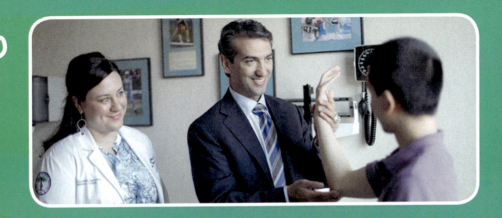

for more information please visit http://www.drahmadsportsmedicine.com/

Final Message from the Authors

While elbow injuries in baseball are a concern, especially for young players, by taking the proper steps of resting, sticking to a reasonable pitch count, and never playing with elbow pain—you can greatly lower your chances of needing Tommy John Surgery. Play smart—and stay healthy on and off the field.

Final Message from the Authors

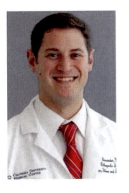

Frank Alexander, MS, ATC

is an athletic trainer at Columbia University Medical Center where he is a part of Dr. Ahmad's clinical staff. He specializes in the care, prevention, and treatment of athletic injuries. As a part of Dr. Ahmad's staff, he helps coordinate the care of many elite athletes such as the New York Yankees, New York City Football Club, Rockland Boulders and many local collegiate and high school athletes.

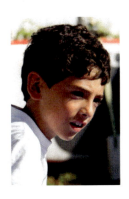

Charles J. Ahmad

is a 7th grade student at Columbia Grammar and Preparatory School, who enjoys computer coding, skiing, playing tennis, and is a tremendous Yankee fan. He has spent time with his father going to the hospital to see patients on weekends and has observed his dad take care of injured athletes and baseball players in the Training Room. He has seen the impact injuries have on athletes and has enjoyed working on this book with his father, and hopes that it will help many young athletes to better understand how to prevent baseball elbow injuries.

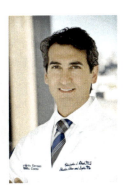

Christopher S. Ahmad, MD

is an orthopedic surgeon at Columbia University Medical Center in New York City. He specializes in shoulder, elbow, and sports medicine injuries. Many of his patients need Tommy John Surgery to get back to playing baseball. Dr. Ahmad is the Head Team Physician for the New York Yankees, New York City Football Club, and Rockland Boulders. He is the acclaimed author of numerous scholarly publications, textbooks, textbook chapters, and books including Skill: 40 Principles that Surgeons, Athletes, and other Elite Performers use to Achieve Mastery.

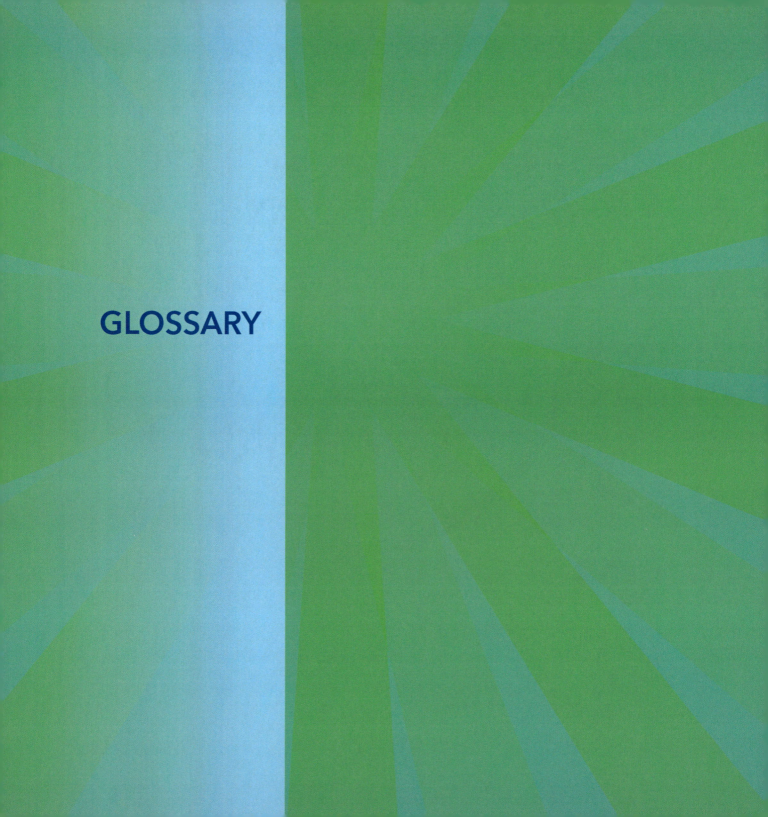
GLOSSARY

Glossary

Athletic Trainer – a health care professional that is an expert at treating, preventing, and educating on athletic injuries.

Bones – any of the pieces of hard, whitish tissue making up the skeleton in humans and other vertebrates.

Dr. Frank Jobe – the doctor that invented the Ulnar Collateral Ligament Reconstruction surgery. The surgery is more famously known as Tommy John Surgery.

Hinged Joint – a joint that allows for two connected bones to move in an L-like range.

Humerus – the upper arm bone.

Ligaments – a short band that connects two bones and holds together a joint.

Medial Epicondyle – a landmark on the humerus that the ulnar collateral ligament originates from.

MRI – a type of imaging a doctor may order so that muscles, tendons, and ligaments can be seen.

Muscles – a group of tissue that can contract (tighten) or relax. Muscles normally work in pairs so you can move your bones in multiple directions.

Nurse – a person trained to care for the sick or infirm, especially in a hospital.

Nurse Practitioner – a nurse who is qualified to treat certain medical conditions without the direct supervision of a doctor.

Olecranon – bump on the back of the elbow that is a part of the ulna.

Orthopedic Doctor – a surgeon who will diagnose their patient and operate on broken bones.

Physical Therapist – restoring movement and reducing pain without surgical treatment.

Pivot Joint – a joint that one bone slides on another, allowing movement.

Radius – bone on the outside of our forearm.

Sublime Tubercle – a landmark on the ulna that the ulnar collateral ligament attaches to.

Symptoms – a physical or mental feature that is regarded as indicating a condition of disease, particularly such a feature that is apparent to the patient.

Tendons – a thick band that attaches muscles to bones.

Tommy John – the baseball player who hurt his Ulnar Collateral Ligament and was the first ever to return from the injury.

UCL Reconstruction Surgery – the surgery that takes a tendon from another part of the patient's body and creates a new ligament so baseball players can throw.

Ulna – bone on the inside of our forearm.

Ulnar Collateral Ligament – the ligament that attaches the ulna and humerus; two of the bones in our arm.

Educational Resources

Dr. Christopher Ahmad's Office – https://www.drahmadsportsmedicine.com

Baseball Health Network – https://baseballhealthnetwork.com/go/

Major League Baseball's Pitch Smart – http://m.mlb.com/pitchsmart/

Made in the USA
Columbia, SC
13 January 2023

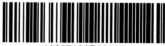